SOLUTION TO CKD

What not to eat and what to eat

Dr. Jack Lucky

TABLE OF CONTENT

INTRODUCTION

"Hope Blooms Here...

Living with Chronic Kidney Disease (CKD) can feel like a dark cloud is following you everywhere. But we want you to know that there is sunshine on the horizon!

In this solution-focused guide, we'll share empowering strategies and nourishing recipes to help you take control of your health and shine brighter than your diagnosis. Our goal is to support you in thriving, not just surviving, with CKD.

Join us on this journey as we explore the power of nutrition, lifestyle changes, and mindful living to transform your health and wellbeing. Let's bloom into a brighter future together!"

Your kidneys perform numerous vital functions. They maintain the balance of your entire body in a number of ways, including:

Eliminating excess water and natural waste from your body

assisting in the production of red blood cells

Maintaining proper mineral balance in your body

assisting with blood pressure maintenance

Maintaining the health of your bones

When the kidneys are unable to perform all of their vital functions due to damage over an extended period of time (at least three months), it is known as chronic kidney disease (CKD). Additionally, heart disease and stroke are among the additional health issues that CKD raises the risk of. The onset of CKD typically occurs gradually and with few symptoms at first. Therefore, the five stages of CKD contribute to inform therapy choices.

SIGNS AND SYMPTOMS

Many CKD patients do not exhibit any symptoms until their condition reaches more advanced stages or until complications arise. If symptoms do appear, they could consist of:

urine with foam

spitting (urinating) more or less frequently than usual

Dry or itchy skin

I'm worn out

emesis

appetite decline

Loss of weight without attempting to reduce
it

Individuals with more severe stages of CKD
could moreover observe:

difficulty focusing

tingling or edema in your legs, ankles, foot,
or arms

cramps or achy muscles

Breathlessness

throwing up

difficulty falling asleep

Ammonia, also referred to as "fishy" or urine-like, is smelled in breath.

CAUSES

Risk factors

CKD can strike anyone, at any age. But some people are more vulnerable than others. The most prevalent risk factors for CKD are:

Diabetes

Hypertension, or elevated blood pressure

Heart failure and/or heart disease

Being overweight

Past the age of sixty

A family history of renal failure or CKD

History of acute kidney injury (AKI) in the individual

either using tobacco goods or smoking

There is often more than one cause of chronic kidney disease (CKD). Rather, a multitude of physical, environmental, and social elements contribute to it. As chronic kidney disease (CKD) frequently starts without any obvious signs, early identification is crucial. Understanding the risk variables can help you determine your level of risk and whether a CKD checkup is necessary.

OTHER CAUSES

CKD can also result from a wide range of other illnesses or situations. Among the instances are:

HIV nephropathy, glomerulonephritis, and IgA nephropathy (IgAN) are examples of glomerular disorders.

Conditions that are inherited: polycystic kidney disease

autoimmune diseases: nephropathy (lupus nephritis)

Severe infections: hemolytic uremic syndrome (HUS) and sepsis

Additional causes include hydronephrosis, kidney and urinary tract anomalies before to birth, kidney cancer, kidney stones, and recurrent, untreated UTIs.

COMPLICATIONS

The likelihood of developing problems increases as CKD develops. Among the instances are:

Heart disease and/or stroke are examples of cardiovascular disease.

elevated blood pressure

Anemia is the low red blood cell count.

Acid accumulation in the blood, or metabolic acidosis

Mineral and bone disorders (resulting in bone and/or heart disease when blood levels of calcium and phosphorus are out of balance)

Hyperkalemia: elevated potassium levels in the blood

renal failure

Cardiovascular disease and high blood pressure are two factors that can aggravate or induce chronic kidney disease (CKD).

DIAGNOSIS

Test

There are two easy tests to check for CKD:

The estimated glomerular filtration rate (eGFR) is a blood test.

a test for albumin-creatinine ratio (uACR) in urine

To get a comprehensive picture of your kidney health, both tests are required. You may have renal disease if your eGFR is less than 60 or your uACR is greater than 30 for three months or longer.

The eGFR is a measure of the kidneys' efficiency in eliminating waste from the blood. It is computed based on your age, sex, and serum creatinine level. You can compute it by utilizing your cystatin C level as well. An eGFR that is considered "normal" changes with age and becomes lower with age. A higher score is desirable for this test. Your CKD stage is ascertained using your eGFR value.

The uACR calculates the concentrations of albumin (a protein) and creatinine in your urine. A healthy kidney filters creatinine out of the urine and maintains albumin in the blood. Therefore, your urine should include either extremely little or no albumin. The amount of urine albumin divided by the amount of urine creatinine yields the ratio, which is used to compute the uACR. In this test, a smaller value is preferable. You can get tested for albuminuria using your uACR value, which is a major risk factor for problems.

To learn more about the condition of your kidneys, your doctor may occasionally prescribe more tests. A kidney biopsy or medical imaging (CT scan, ultrasound, or MRI) are a couple of examples.

TREATMENT FOR CKD

Overview The four main objectives of managing CKD are as follows:

Taking care of the ailment or conditions—such as diabetes, high blood pressure, or IgA nephropathy—that are most likely the source of your chronic kidney disease (CKD).

Taking action to directly slow down the course of the CKD disease (sometimes referred to as "slowing CKD progression").
reducing the chance of developing cardiovascular disease (heart attack or stroke)
addressing any CKD-related issues you may be experiencing
Your CKD stage and any coexisting medical illnesses (including consequences from your CKD) will determine the specific course of treatment that is recommended for you. The guidelines listed below are applicable to the majority of CKD patients. Since no two people are alike, discuss recommendations made specifically for you with your healthcare provider.

MEDICATIONS

To help slow down or stop the progression of your CKD, your healthcare provider may prescribe one or more medications. These medications may consist of nsMRAs, SGLT2 inhibitors, and/or ACE inhibitors/ARBs.

A statin, or cholesterol medication, may also be recommended by your medical practitioner. According to guidelines, anyone with CKD who also have diabetes, a history of heart disease, or who are 50 years of age or older should take a statin. A statin can help reduce your risk of heart attack or stroke even if you do not have high cholesterol.

In order to treat any potential consequences from your CKD, you might additionally need to take extra drugs or vitamins (if relevant).

NUTRITION

It's crucial to keep your daily consumption of sodium, or salt, to less than 2300 mg, or around one teaspoon from all the food and beverages you eat and drink. In the event that you also have high blood pressure, this advice is crucial. A lower target may be recommended by your healthcare provider based on your other medical concerns. This is much more than just not using a saltshaker; it also entails avoiding foods that have high sodium content shown on the nutrition facts label. If you read the nutrition information label on a food that doesn't taste salty, you might be surprised to learn how much sodium it contains.

Your doctor or kidney dietician may also suggest that you adjust your dietary intake of potassium, phosphorus, and/or calcium in light of the findings of your blood tests.

Seeking advice from a nutritionist can be particularly beneficial if you already suffer from other medical issues such as high blood pressure, diabetes, or heart failure. In these cases, including a nutritious diet into your daily routine is even more crucial in preventing complications. Keeping track of so many changes might be difficult, but a nutritionist can help you figure out what suits you the best.

Visit the Nutrition and Early Kidney Disease website for more details on eating well when you have kidney disease.

LIFESTYLE RECOMMENDATIONS

This is an excellent moment to adopt a healthy lifestyle:

Give up smoking and/or using tobacco products. Smoking raises your risk of developing renal failure and accelerates the course of kidney disease. It also raises your risk for heart disease, cancer, stroke, high blood pressure, and other major health issues.
Engage in regular exercise. Recall that starting out slowly is acceptable; taking quick walks is a terrific place to start.

Getting enough sleep is also essential. In order to be well-rested, try to obtain adequate sleep.

Losing weight with exercise and a balanced diet can help improve your health in many ways if you are overweight.

Look for strategies to handle and lessen stress in your life.

OTHER WAYS TO LOWER YOUR RISK

Managing any additional medical conditions you may have can also benefit your chronic kidney disease (CKD). excessive blood pressure, diabetes, and excessive cholesterol are examples of this.

Non-steroid anti-inflammatory drugs (NSAIDs) are a class of painkillers that people with chronic kidney disease (CKD) should stay away from. Your kidneys may be harmed by them, particularly if you use them frequently or at greater dosages. Among the instances are:

ibuprofen (Advil, Motrin)
indocin (indomethacin)
naproxen (Naprosyn, Aleve)
diclofenac pills or capsules (Zipsor, Cataflam)
Meloxicam (Mobic) with celecoxib (Celebrex)
aspirin (but only up to 325 mg daily)
Many of these over-the-counter (OTC) NSAID medications are accessible; they might be marketed differently or combined with other medications (such as cough and cold remedies). Depending on your other medical conditions, using these products might not always be avoidable. Before utilizing any items with these drug names or if the product label has the word "NSAID," always consult your healthcare provider. When taken as directed, acetaminophen, often known as Tylenol, is generally safe for your kidneys. However, consult a healthcare

provider to find the source of your pain and the most effective course of action.

Increasing your daily intake of fruits and vegetables can help lower the level of acid in your blood if your healthcare provider diagnoses you with metabolic acidosis. This may also assist in delaying the worsening of your CKD.

NUTRITION AND CHRONIC KIDNEY DISEASE

Kidney disease can be slowed down in its progression by eating the appropriate meals and avoiding the bad ones. You can create an eating plan that is appropriate for your stage of chronic renal disease with the assistance of a qualified dietitian.

Sodium

Numerous foods naturally contain the mineral sodium. You are adding sodium to your diet when you use table salt.

The kidneys' normal ability to remove excess salt is compromised by kidney disease. This results in an imbalance between salt and water in your body, which can cause high blood pressure, excessive thirst, and swelling of your hands, feet, and face.

Calcium
One mineral that is crucial to the operation of your heart is potassium. Excess or insufficient potassium levels can lead to serious health complications.2.

Too high or too low potassium levels might result from kidney disease. If your potassium levels are excessively high, your doctor could suggest reducing your intake of foods high in potassium. You might need to eat more of these items when they're too low.3.

phosphorus

Your bones may become weaker as a result of low calcium levels brought on by high phosphorus levels. Additionally, they may result in the accumulation of calcium in your heart, lungs, and blood vessels, among other areas of your body.

Your chance of suffering a heart attack or stroke may rise as a result.4
Depending on your stage of renal illness, you will require a different diet. For example, you will need to reduce salt in the early stages. To maintain your blood levels within acceptable ranges in later phases, you might also need to restrict your intake of potassium and/or phosphorus.5. You must consume high-quality protein from foods like meat, poultry, fish, and eggs while receiving dialysis.Six

FOODS TO AVOID

It's crucial to alter your diet to assist decrease the illness's progression and enhance your general health and well-being, regardless of the stage of kidney disease you've been diagnosed with.

Certain foods are frequently restricted or avoided by patients with renal disease, including:

complete grains
Granola, oatmeal, and bran cereals
Sunflower seeds and nuts
Avocado Tomatoes
Some more fruits, both fresh and dried (bananas, apricots, etc.)
Milk
Sweet potatoes
legumes
Beet greens, spinach, and Swiss chard
Chips, pretzels, and crackers
Pickles and sauce
meats that have been processed
meals that are prepared or frozen

Foods in cans
sodas with a dark color
Complete Grains
Although whole grains contain more potassium and phosphorus than refined grains, they are still frequently advised for those without kidney problems. Your healthcare professional could suggest avoiding whole grain foods like brown rice and whole wheat bread if you have moderate to advanced renal disease.

For instance, 28 grams (or one slice) of whole grain bread contains: 7

69 milligrams or so of potassium
57 milligrams of phosphorus
Comparatively, a white bread slice of the same size contains: 8

32.8 milligrams of potassium
31.6 milligrams of P
A cooked cup of brown rice yields approximately 9.

208 mg of potassium and 174 mg of phosphorous

Comparatively, 10 grams of cooked white rice make approximately 1 cup.

54 mg of potassium and 69 mg of phosphorus

Bran Granola, oatmeal, and cereal

Make sure to read the product label while purchasing both hot and cold cereals. There are a lot of cereals at the grocery shop that contain:

Sodium Phosphorus

Calcium

Céréales with additional phosphorus should be limited or avoided. Phosphorus, often known as "phos," isn't needed to be listed on the Nutrition Facts label like potassium and sodium are, so look for it in the ingredients list. About 11 grams make approximately 3/4 cup of bran flakes cereal.

160 milligrams of potassium
A 135 mg phosphorus dose
When cooked oatmeal is cup, it contains: 12

180 mg of potassium and 164 mg of phosphorous
Oats are used to make most granola. Granola is generally a healthy choice, but because it contains potassium, it should be consumed in moderation when following a renal diet.

About 306 milligrams of potassium may be found in two ounces of granola.Thirteen

Nuts and seeds of sunflowers
For most individuals, nuts and seeds make popular and healthful snacks. However, they may be dangerous for someone who has kidney disease.

One ounce, or roughly 23 almonds, makes up about 14

208 milligrams of potassium

136 mg of phosphorus in cashews is approximately 15

Potassium, 187 mg

168 milligrams of P

If you're a fan of nuts and sunflower seeds, think about having them with other meals that are low in phosphorus and potassium. As an alternative, go for nuts with less phosphorous.

Tomatoes Potassium content is high in tomatoes. It is typically not necessary for people with renal disease in its early stages to restrict their tomato intake. But tomatoes could have to be on your limited foods list if your doctor says your potassium levels are excessive.

This covers tomato-based goods like sauce and ketchup as well as raw tomatoes.

For instance, 910 mg of potassium can be found in one cup of tomato sauce.16 About 292 mg of potassium are found in one medium tomato.17

Avocados
Avocados are a fantastic source of essential vitamins and minerals as well as heart-healthy lipids. But since they contain a lot of potassium, they shouldn't be consumed while on a renal diet.

There are roughly 690 mg of potassium in one avocado.18

You should avoid or consume guacamole and avocados in moderation if your healthcare physician has advised you to restrict your potassium intake.

Some Other Fruits
Certain fruits have a lot of potassium. If your kidney doctor or nutritionist has

advised you to limit your potassium consumption, you should stay away from:

One of the healthiest foods to include in your diet is bananas. There are an astounding 422 mg of potassium in one medium banana.19 Oranges have a lot of potassium as well. About 255 mg of potassium20 are found in one orange, while 443 mg are found in one cup of orange juice.21

Apricots: Apricots should be avoided in advanced kidney illness due to their potassium concentration. 427 milligrams of potassium can be found in one cup of sliced apricots.22

Dried fruits may also provide issues. Raisins and prunes, in addition to dried apricots, are rich in calories, sugar, and potassium. Around 1,510 milligrams of potassium can be found in one cup of dried apricots. This easily meets your recommended daily amount of potassium.

Furthermore, 1,270 mg of potassium can be found in one cup of prunes.23 In its unprocessed form, the potassium is somewhat lower nevertheless. Just 259 milligrams of potassium are found in one cup of plums.24

Dairy Products Rich sources of calcium, protein, and other essential nutrients include cheese, yogurt, milk, and ice cream. They also contain a lot of potassium and phosphorus.

A patient with advanced renal illness may need to restrict their intake of protein, phosphorus, and potassium, which will also require them to cut back on dairy.

In one cup of 2% milk, there are 25

Eight grammes of protein
390 mg of potassium and 252 mg of phosphorous

Potatoes: By nature, potatoes are rich in potassium. About 610 mg of potassium can be found in one medium potato.26

Thankfully, there are methods for lowering the potassium level in potatoes. Leaching potatoes (soaking them in water) is one of the greatest techniques to reduce their potassium level before cooking.

Boiling the potatoes for around ten minutes while they are sliced into little pieces is the most efficient approach to extract potassium through leaching. By doing this, the potassium content can be lowered to at least half its initial value.27

Beans: Beans are a fantastic source of fiber and plant-based protein. If you eat them in big amounts, though, they can also raise the levels of potassium and phosphorus in your blood.28

Recent research suggests that those with chronic renal disease can benefit from eating beans and legumes as a source of protein.29 Guidelines however advise against consuming too many beans because of their high potassium and phosphorus content.

As an illustration, one cup of cooked pinto beans has 746 mg of potassium and 251 mg of phosphorus.30

Beet greens, spinach, and Swiss Chard
Because of their high potassium level, the majority of leafy green vegetables—including spinach, beet greens, and Swiss chard—are not advised on a diet for kidney illness.

For instance, 839 mg of potassium is included in one cup of cooked spinach, which is about half of the daily requirement for someone with high potassium levels and chronic renal disease.31

Chips, Pretzels, and Crackers
Salt content is often high in snack items like pretzels, chips, and crackers. They also lack vital nutrients that your body requires in order to function correctly.

Since potato chips are made from potatoes, they should be avoided as they are also high in potassium.

Approximately 150 mg of salt and 336 mg of potassium are present in one small bag of potato chips (22 chips).32

Pickles and Sauce
Curried foods include relish and pickles. They should be avoided on a renal diet due to their high sodium content.

One large pickle, for instance, has about 1,630 mg of sodium in it. A person following a kidney-friendly diet is typically advised to limit their daily sodium intake to 2,300 mg.33

Prepared Meats
Meats that have been fermented, smoked, salted, or cured in order to enhance flavor and prolong shelf life are referred to as processed meats.

Processed meats include things like pepperoni, hot dogs, sausage, beef jerky, and corned beef.

Consuming red and processed meats raises the risk of developing chronic kidney disease.34

Processed meat has a high protein content in addition to a high salt content.
Prepared or Thawed Food
The majority of processed foods, such as frozen or prepared meals, are heavy in sodium. Soups, frozen pizza, and premade frozen dinners are a few examples.

Premade meals should be avoided when following a kidney diet, as they often contain the majority of the daily sodium intake that is advised.

Foods in Cans

Soups, vegetables, meats, and seafood are among the many items that are popularly canned since they are an easy and quick way to increase the amount of nutrient-rich foods in your diet.

But because salt is frequently added to canned foods as a preservative to increase their shelf life, the majority of them are high in sodium.

Canned foods should be avoided because a person with chronic renal disease cannot eliminate excess salt.35 Sodas in Dark Colors

The majority of dark-colored sodas use a lot of phosphorus additions to lengthen their shelf lives and improve their flavor. They should be restricted on all diets due to their high sugar and calorie content.

A 200 milliliter serving of most dark-colored sodas has 50–100 mg of phosphorus in it.36

Research indicates that phosphorus supplements are more quickly absorbed than phosphorus found in plants or the environment.37

One exception is root beer, which has less than one milligram of potassium and phosphorus per serving.38

1. Blueberries Rich in minerals and antioxidants called anthocyanins, blueberries may offer protection against diabetes, heart disease, and other illnesses (Trusted Source).

They also have low potassium, phosphorus, and salt contents.

Fresh blueberries weigh 148 grams (one cup) and containReliable Source:

Protein: 1 g; sodium: 1.5 mg; potassium: 114 mg; phosphorus: 18 mg

2. Sea bass High-quality protein can be obtained from sea bass. Additionally, it has omega-3s, which are good fats. Omega-3 fatty acids have the potential to improve long-term condition patients' health and prevent a variety of ailments (Trusted Source).

Three ounces (eighty-five grams) of cooked sea bass hasReliable Source:

74 milligrams of sodium
20 g of protein, 279 mg of potassium, and 211 mg of phosphorus

3. Grapes in red color

Flavonoids, an antioxidant class of antioxidants found in red grapes, may help lower inflammation and offer protection against heart disease, diabetes, and other illnesses.

75 grams, or half a cup, of red grapesReliable Source:

Protein: 0.5 g5, sodium: 1.5 mg, potassium: 144 mg, and phosphorus: 15 mg.

4.White eggs
Low in phosphorus and high in quality, egg whites are a kidney-friendly source of protein.

Given that egg yolks can contain significant levels of phosphorus, egg whites may be a better option than whole eggs for those following a renal diet.

Two substantial, uncooked egg whites (66 g) haveReliable Source:

110 milligrams of sodium
Protein: 7 g; Potassium: 108 mg; Phosphorus: 10 mg

5. Onion
Garlic adds taste to food and has nutritional advantages, making it a delicious substitute for salt.

It's a good source of B6 and manganese. Additionally, it has anti-inflammatory sulfur compounds from a trusted source.

Nine grams (three cloves) of garlic containReliable Source:

Protein: 0.5 g, sodium: 1.5 mg, potassium: 36 mg, and phosphorus: 14 mg.

6. Buckwheat

One entire grain that is low in potassium is buckwheat. In addition, it has fiber, iron, magnesium, and B vitamins.

Additionally, it is free of gluten, making it appropriate for those who have a gluten sensitivity or celiac disease.

Half a cup, or 85 grams, of buckwheat hasReliable Source:

0.8 mg of sodium, 391 mg of potassium, 295 mg of phosphorus, and 11 g of protein.

7.Olive oil
Olive oil is primarily composed of unsaturated fat and is a good source of vitamin E. Additionally, it has no phosphorus, which makes it a good choice for those who have renal illness.

Oleic acid, which makes up the majority of the fat in olive oil, has anti-inflammatory qualities (Trusted Source).

Additionally stable at high temperatures are monounsaturated fats like olive oil, which makes it a healthy option for cooking.

A tablespoon's worth (14 g) of olive oilReliable Source:

Protein: 0 g; sodium: 0.3 mg; potassium: 0.1 mg; and phosphorus: 0 mg.

8. Bulgur
A whole grain product made of wheat, bulgur is a kidney-friendly substitute for other whole grains that include greater levels of phosphorus and potassium.

Bulgur offers plant-based protein and fiber, which are crucial for digestive health, along with B vitamins, iron, and magnesium.

When cooked, a half-cup (70 g) portion of bulgur includesReliable Source:

154 milligrams of sodium
48 mg of potassium, 28 mg of phosphorus, and 2 g of protein.

9.Broccoli
A member of the cruciferous vegetable family, cabbage is high in antioxidants, vitamins, and minerals.

A study's authors from 2021According to Trusted Source, red, green, and white cabbage can be beneficial:

control your blood sugar
lower the chance of liver and kidney damage
prevent obesity and oxidative stress
Shredded savoy cabbage in a cup (70 g) includesReliable Source:

20 milligrams of sodium
Protein: 1.4 g; potassium: 161 mg; phosphorus: 29 mg 11.

10.Compared to chicken with the skin on, skinless chicken breasts are lower in fat and phosphorus.

Cooked, skinless chicken breast weighed one cup (140 g) and containedReliable Source:

43 g of protein, 104 mg of sodium, 358 mg of potassium, and 319 mg of phosphorus. NIDDK recommends Trusted People who suffer from renal illness should only eat 2-3 ounces of meat or fish each day because eating too much protein might strain the kidneys.

11. Peppers with bells
Bell peppers are low in potassium but high in antioxidants such as vitamins A and C.

The immune system, which is strongly associated with kidney disease, depends on these nutrients.

One hundred grams (100 g) of medium red peppers contains

Less than 2.5 mg of sodium, 213 mg of potassium, 27 mg of phosphorus, and 1 g of protein 13.

12.Onions
Onions are one way to give dishes on the renal diet taste without adding sodium, even if reducing salt might be difficult.

You may flavor food without endangering your kidneys by sautéing onions with garlic, olive oil, and herbs.

Vitamin C, manganese, and B vitamins, including folate, are all found in onions. Additionally, they contain prebiotic fibers from Trusted Source, which support healthy gut flora and aid in maintaining the health of your digestive system.

A 70 g little onion has the following contents: Reliable Source:

3 mg of sodium
Protein: 0.8 g; potassium: 102 mg; phosphorus: 20 mg

CONCLUSION

"You Did It!

Congratulations on taking the first steps towards a brighter, healthier future! By embracing the solutions and strategies in this guide, you've shown that you're committed to thriving, not just surviving, with CKD.

Remember, every small change adds up to make a big difference. You've got this! You are stronger than your diagnosis, and you deserve to live a life filled with purpose, joy, and vitality.

Keep shining, keep thriving, and know that you're not alone on this journey. You've got a community of warriors cheering you on every step of the way!

To a healthier, happier you - and a brighter future ahead!"
THE END

www.ingramcontent.com/pod-product-compliance
Lightning Source LLC
Chambersburg PA
CBHW051714250726
48653CB00007B/3017